MR. BAD BUG!

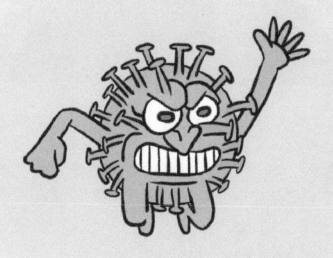

Mr. Bad Bug

Published by Gatekeeper Press
2167 Stringtown Rd, Suite 109
Columbus, OH 43123-2989
www.GatekeeperPress.com

Library of Congress Control Number: 2020946092

ISBN (hardcover): 9781662904653
ISBN (paperback): 9781662904660
ISBN: 9781662904677

MR. BAD BUG!

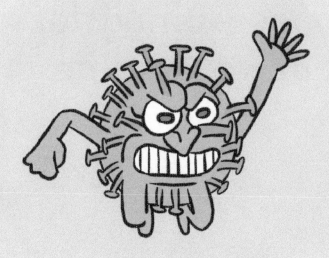

Giannis Charonis
Sia Charonis
Nicholas Charonis

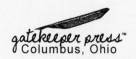
gatekeeper press™
Columbus, Ohio

Mr. Bad Bug, we've heard about you.

Everyone's waiting to see what you will do.

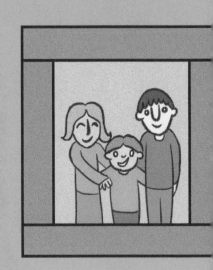

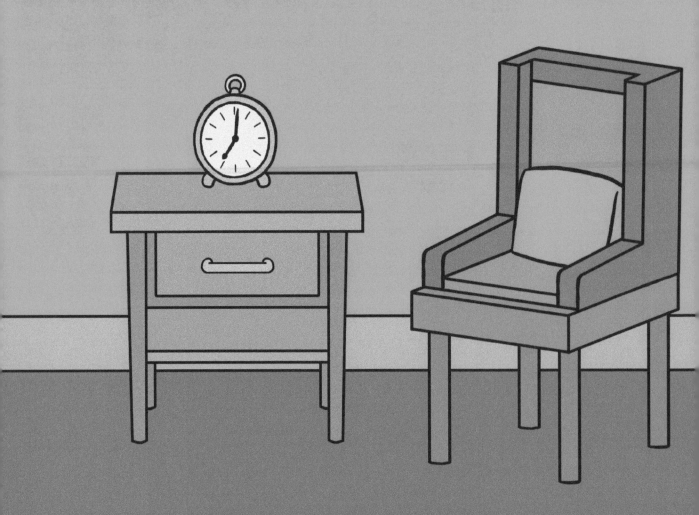

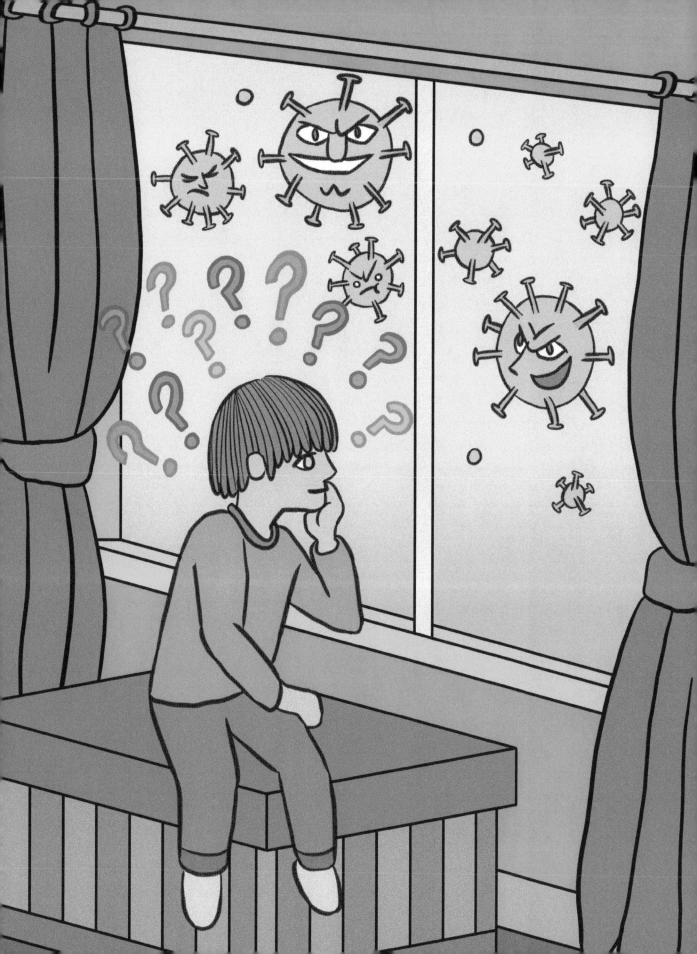

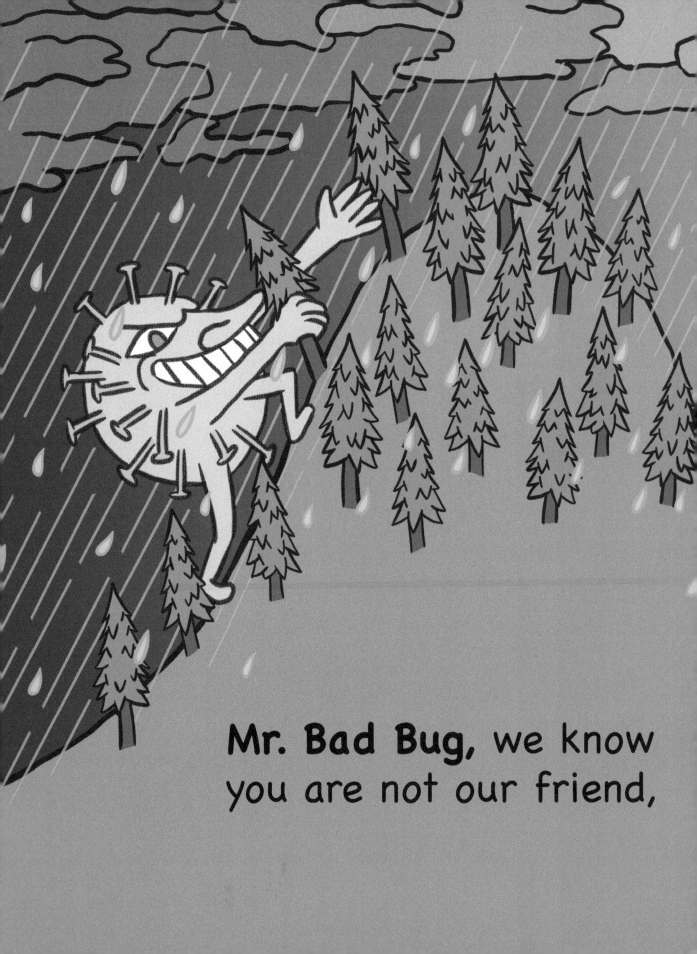

Mr. Bad Bug, we know
you are not our friend,

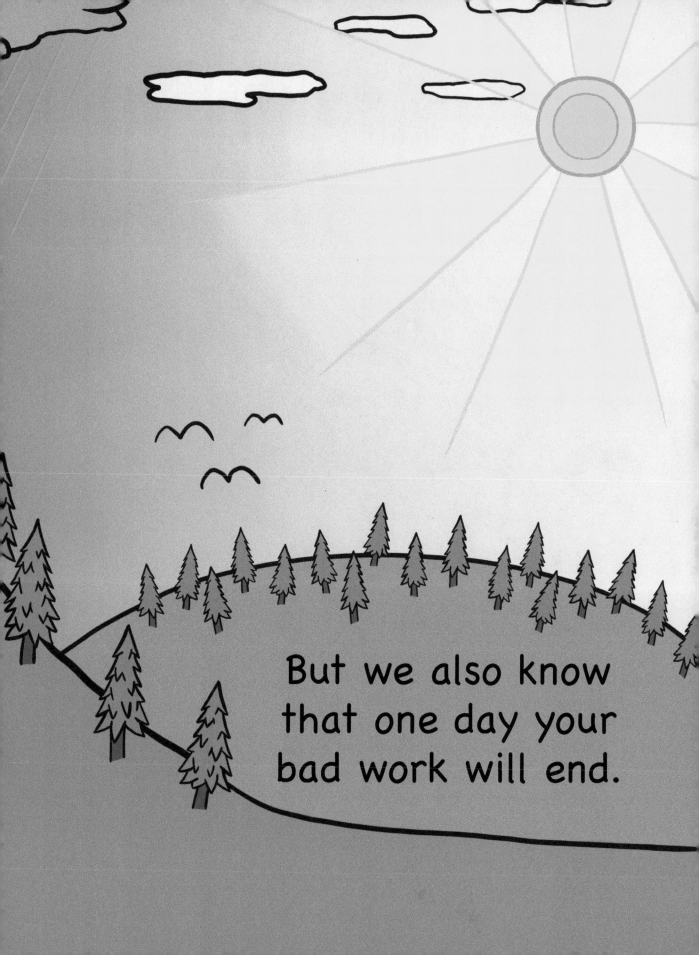

But we also know
that one day your
bad work will end.

Mr. Bad Bug, until then we will be strong,

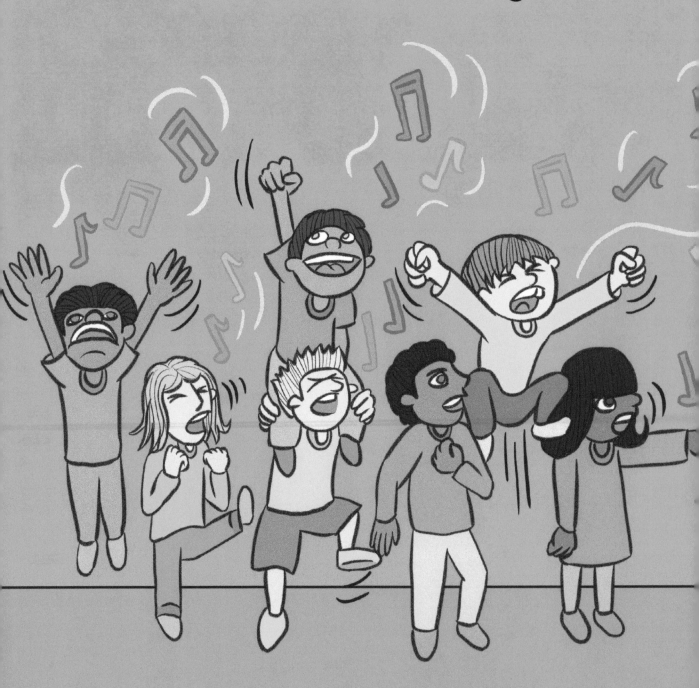

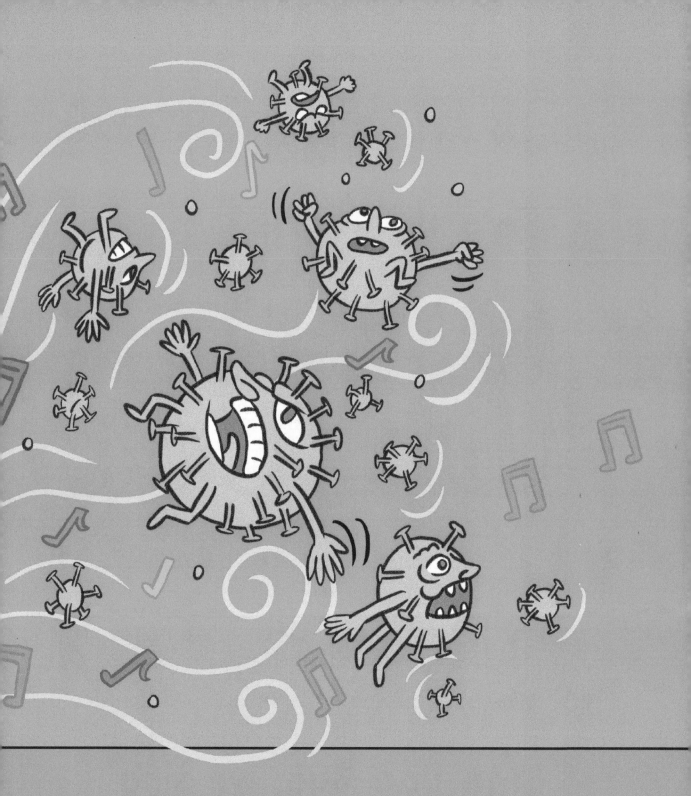

And keep our spirits up
with a daily song.

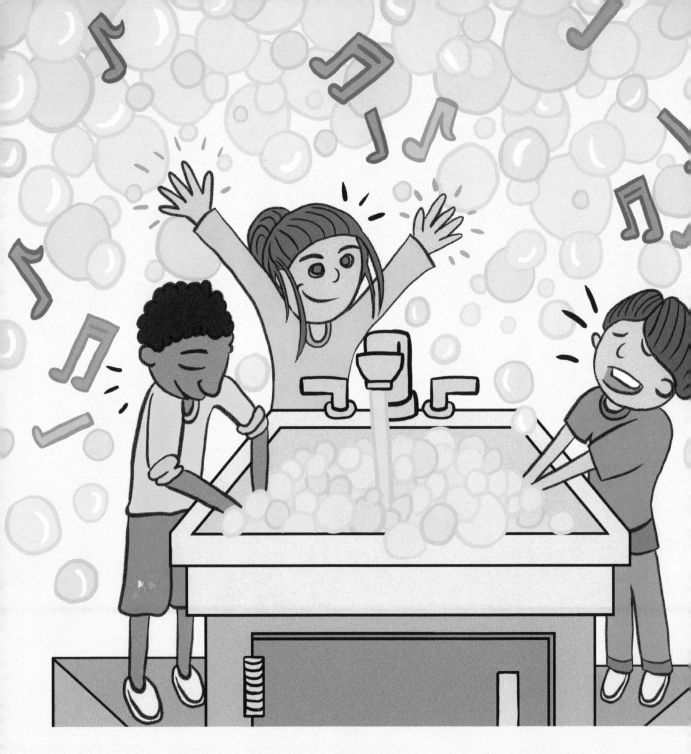

Mr. Bad Bug, we sing
our alphabet as we
wash our hands,

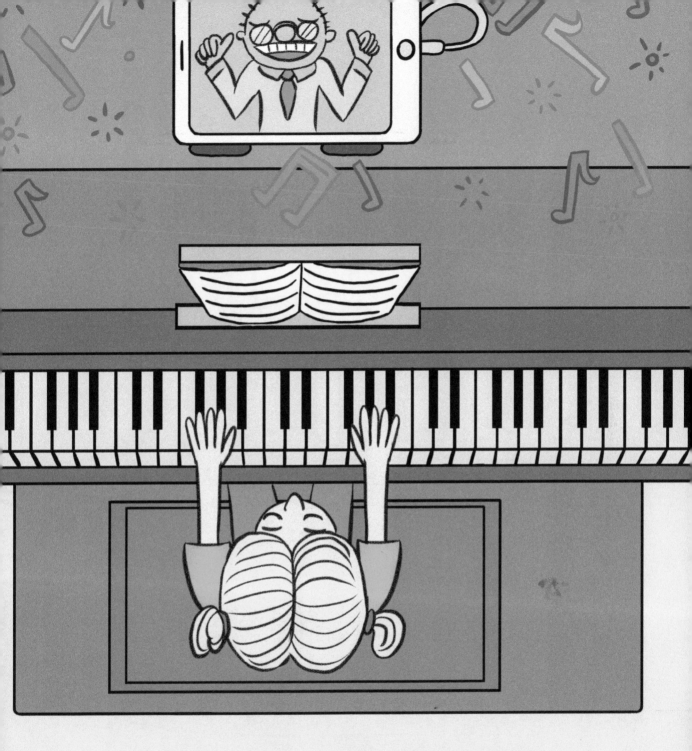

And we still do music lessons remotely with iPad stands.

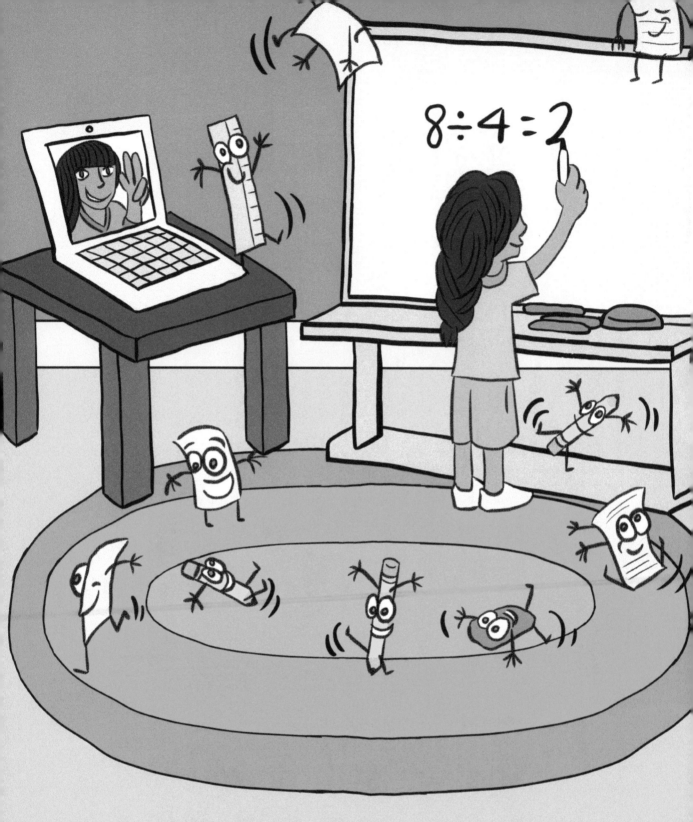

Mr. Bad Bug, you can't stop us from learning.

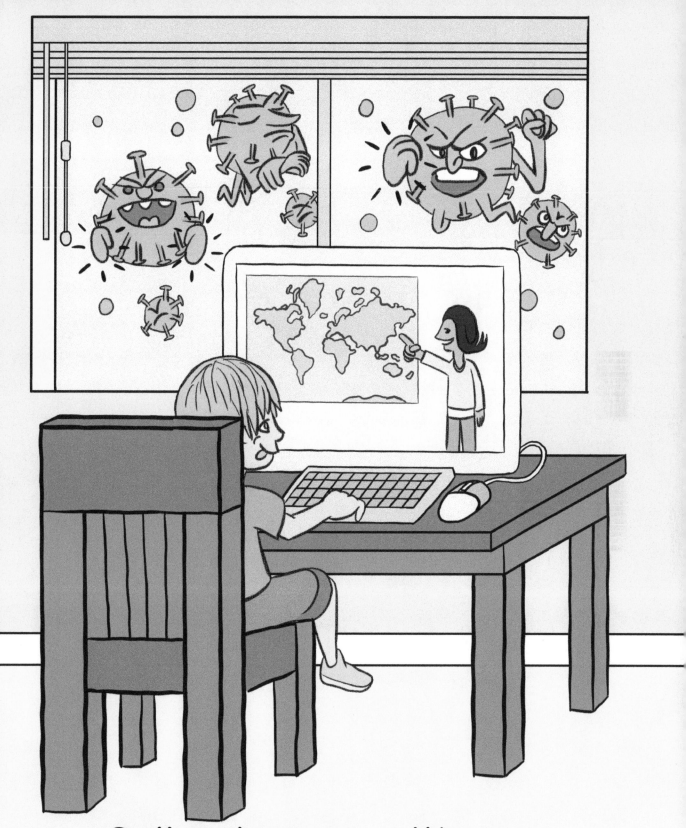

Online lessons with our
teachers aren't concerning.

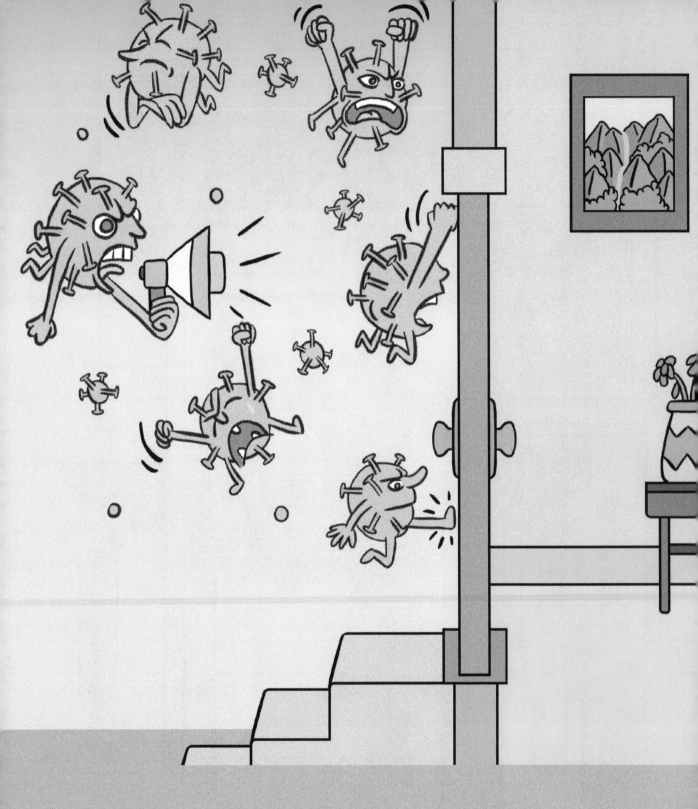

Mr. Bad Bug, you have
kept us all inside,

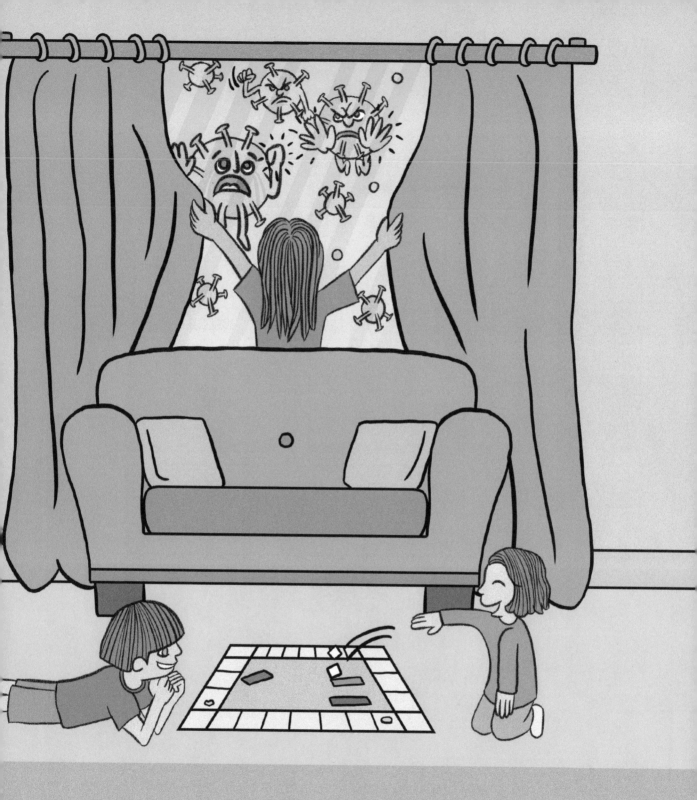

But we still play indoors
and keep our pride!

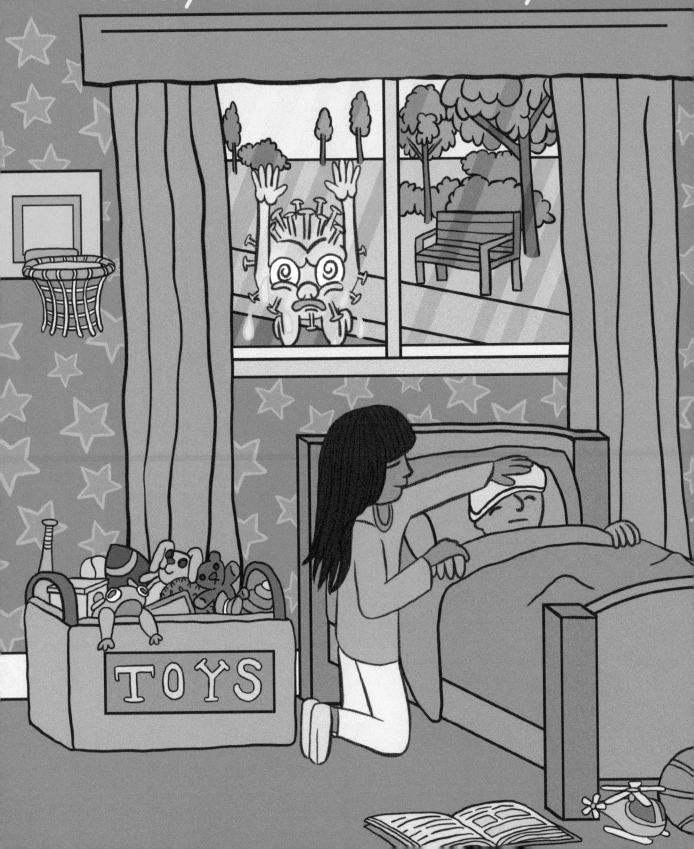

Mr. Bad Bug, some people are really sick because of you.

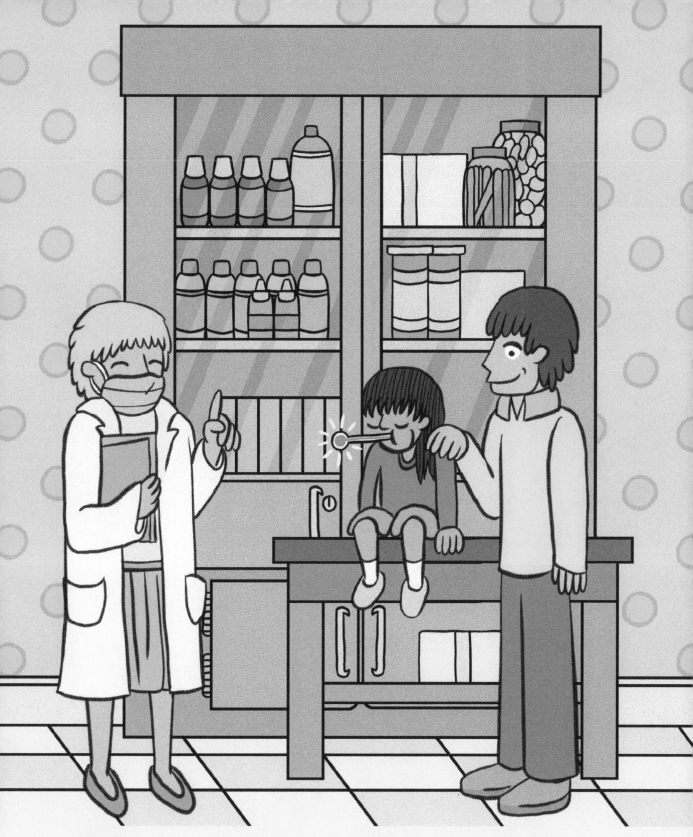

Some people need medicine
because they are feeling blue.

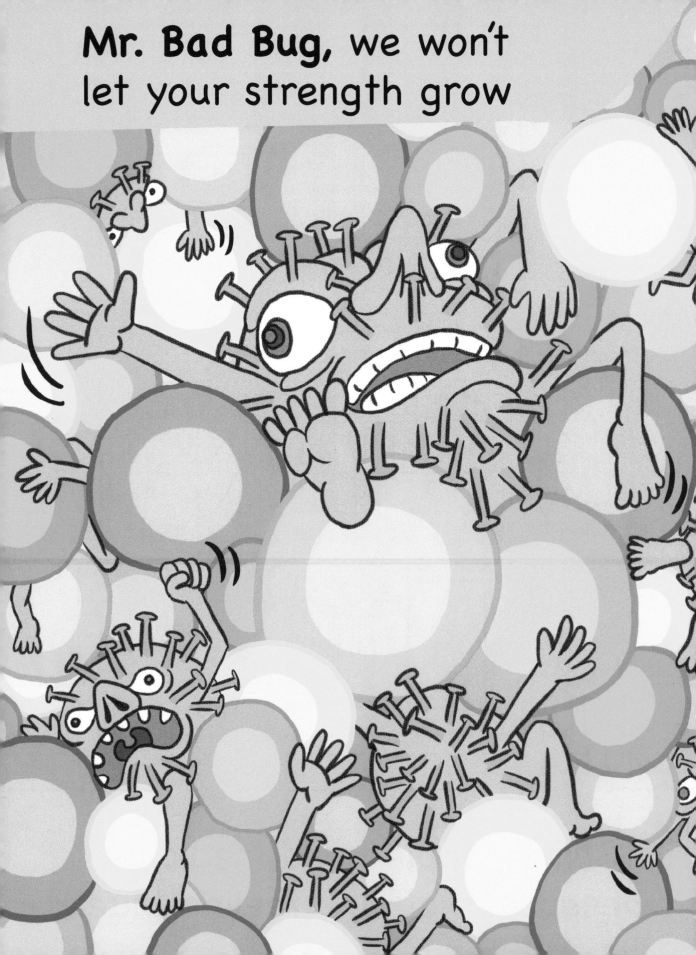

Mr. Bad Bug, we won't let your strength grow

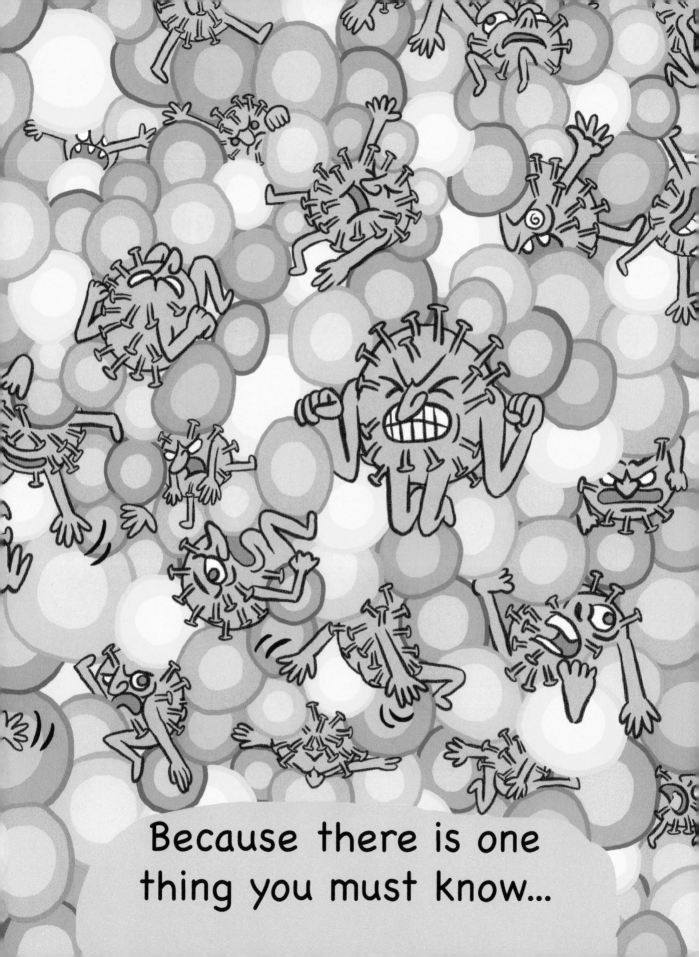

Because there is one
thing you must know...

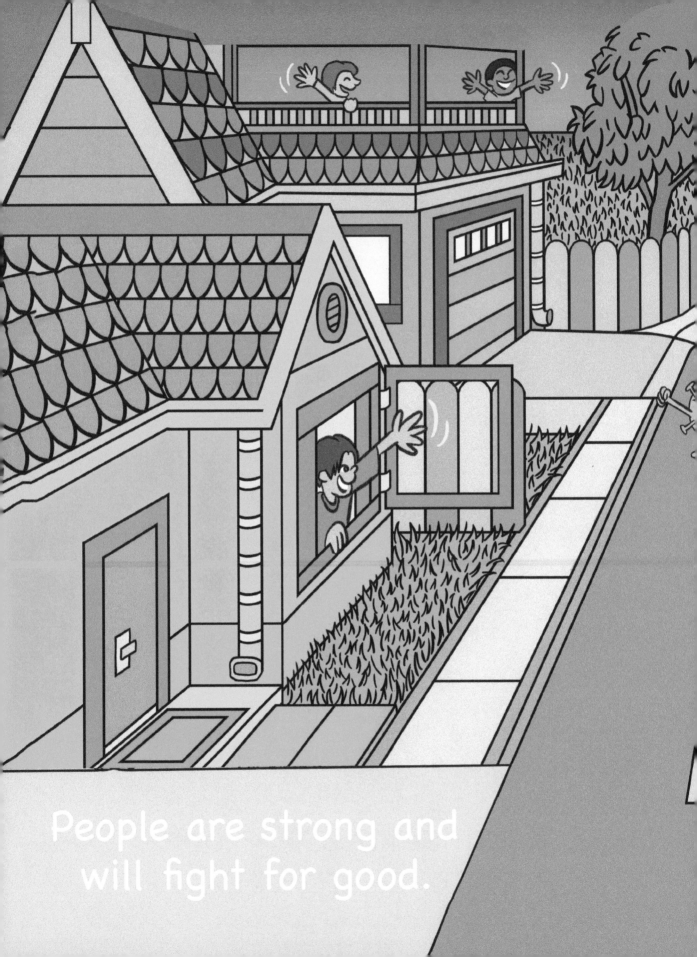

People are strong and
will fight for good.

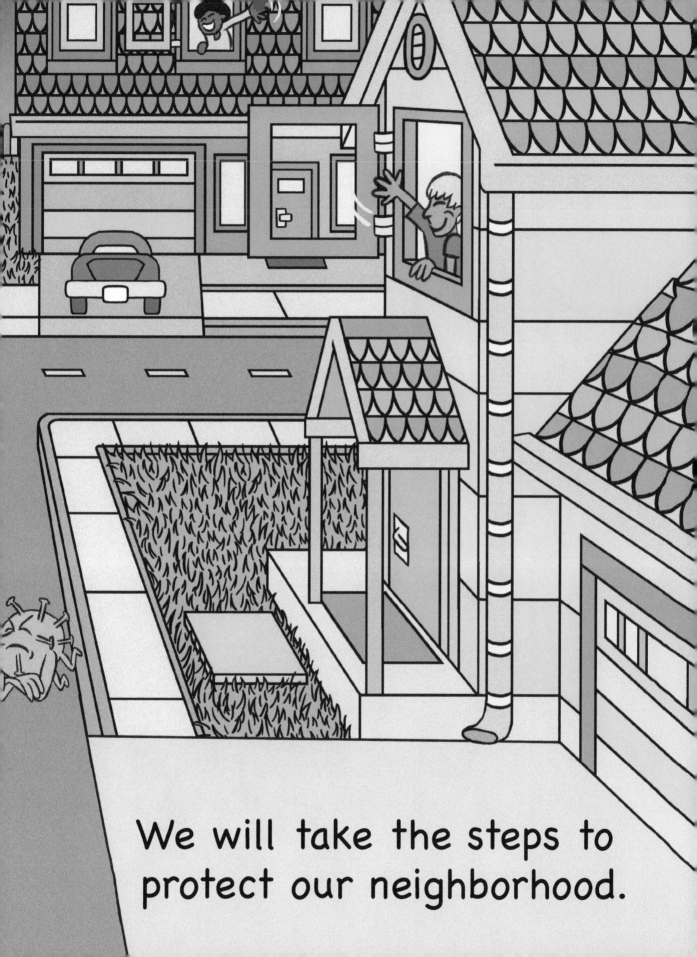

We will take the steps to protect our neighborhood.

Mr. **Bad Bug,** we will not go too close to others.

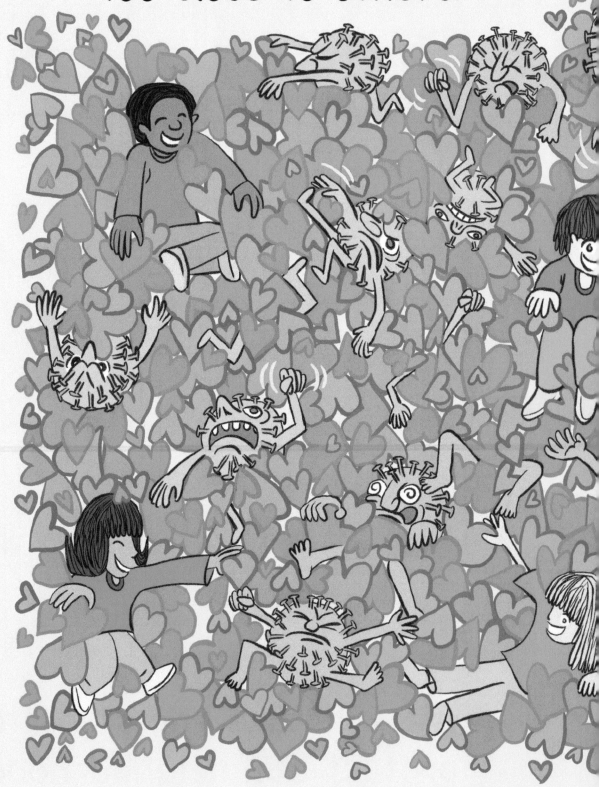

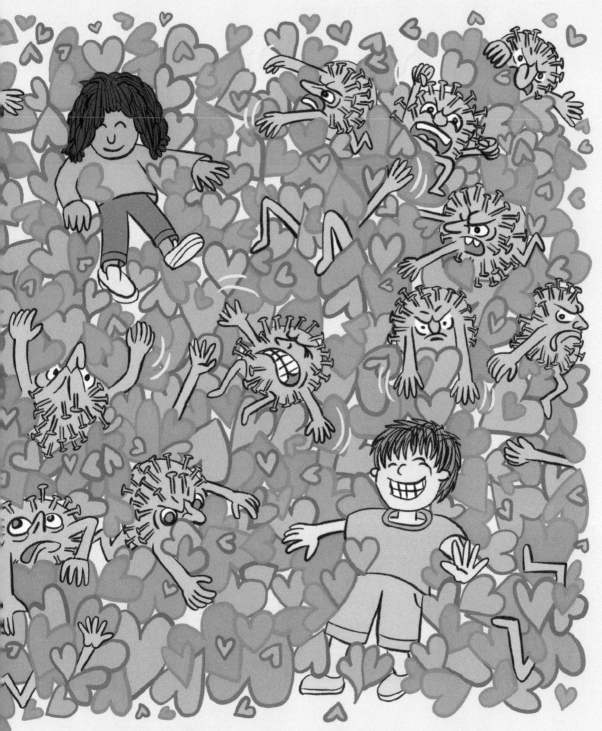

We will be extra safe -
not just for us, but for our
sisters and brothers.

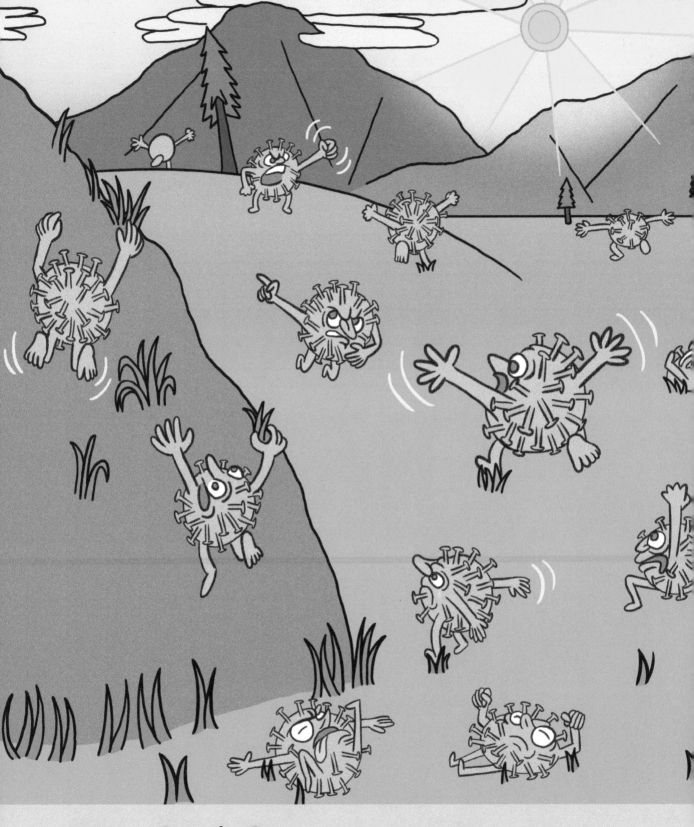

Mr. Bad Bug, when we have
sent you far away,

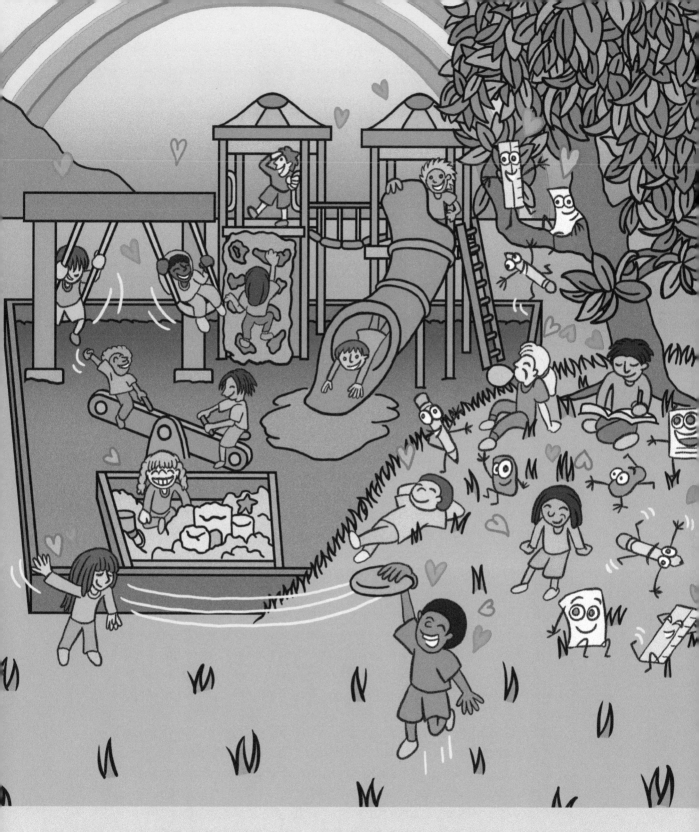

We will go outside once more
for another beautiful day!

About the Authors

Giannis Charonis is a 10 year old 5th grader who came up with the original idea of "Mr. Bad Bug." The idea came to him when explaining to his younger siblings why they couldn't go out and play with their friends like the "old days" during the Corona Virus pandemic. Mr. Bad Bug turned into a short poem Giannis created. He shared Mr. Bad Bug with his class and it soon became a household explanation for why his siblings and cousins couldn't do some of the things they were used to. Seeing how well the younger children took to the concept of "Mr. Bad Bug" as a "matter of fact" explanation that they easily understood, Giannis, working with his mother, decided to try and find a way to bring this story to children around the globe and make it easier for them all to understand the global pandemic, and "bad bugs" generally.

Sia Charonis is a mother of 2 boys Giannis (10) and Vasili (5), and one daughter Stella (3). When she's not busy as a full time tech attorney in Silicon Valley, she's otherwise looking for ways to keep her energetic children occupied and embracing all this world has to offer. The recent global Corona Virus pandemic was an opportunity for her to teach her children more about the "bad bugs" that are out there, why typical daily routines had to be adjusted and to help remain focused on positivity. Sia wanted to help turn what could be a scary situation into one that could be understood through the eyes of a child by helping her son Giannis turn his short poem on Mr. Bad Bug into a children's book.

Nicholas Charonis is Giannis' cousin and an up and coming graphic designer. When he heard the story of Mr. Bad Bug he helped use his amazing talents to bring colorful life to the words on the pages. Nicholas uses digital art and metaphoric graphics to take readers on a colorful journey of Mr. Bad Bug, giving hope and positivity that there is beauty in this world both with and without Mr. Bad Bug around!